THE WOMEN'S GUIDE TO OPTIMAL NUTRITION

Nourishing Your Body and Mind

A.C. Stallings RN

independent

ISBN-13: 9798854869058

Cover design by: Art Painter
Library of Congress Control Number: 2018675309
Printed in the United States of America

INTRODUCTION

In today's fast-paced world, women have a lot on their plates. That's why it's crucial for them to prioritize their well-being, starting with nutrition. Good nutrition is essential at every stage of life, from adolescence to pregnancy and menopause. It's what fuels women's bodies, empowering them to live fulfilling lives and reach their goals.

When women feed their bodies with the right nutrients, amazing things happen. Energy levels soar, immune function is boosted, and the risk of chronic diseases decreases. But it's not just about staying healthy - it's about thriving.

Imagine having the energy to tackle your to-do list, manage your responsibilities, and still have some left in the tank for yourself. By incorporating nutrient-rich foods into your diet, you can supercharge your productivity, mood, and overall well-being.

It's time to take control of your nutrition and unleash your potential. Invest in yourself and reap the benefits that women's nutrition brings to your body and mind.

Table of Contents

THE WOMEN'S GUIDE TO OPTIMAL NUTRITION: NOURISHING YOUR BODY AND MIND

CHAPTER 1: UNDERSTANDING WOMEN'S NUTRITION

The Importance of Women's Nutrition

In today's fast-paced world, women must prioritize their overall well-being, and one key aspect of this is nutrition. Proper nutrition plays a vital role in supporting women's health, allowing them to lead fulfilling lives and achieve their goals. This subchapter emphasizes the significance of women's nutrition and highlights the various benefits it brings to their bodies and minds.

Good nutrition is essential for women at every stage of life, from adolescence to pregnancy and menopause. It is through a well-balanced diet that women can fuel their bodies with the nutrients to maintain optimal health. Adequate nutrition offers several advantages, including

improved energy levels, enhanced immune function, and a reduced risk of chronic diseases.

Women's nutrition increases energy levels, which is one of its primary benefits. Proper nourishment provides the body with the fuel it needs to function efficiently. Women often lead busy lives, juggling various responsibilities, and a well-nourished body can help maintain their energy levels throughout the day. By incorporating nutrient-rich foods into their diet, women can enhance their productivity and overall well-being.

Optimal nutrition plays a crucial role in supporting a healthy immune system. Women are often more susceptible to infections and illnesses, and a well-balanced diet can help strengthen their immune response. Key nutrients like vitamins A, C, and E, as well as zinc and selenium, are vital for maintaining a robust immune system. By consuming a variety of fruits, vegetables, lean proteins, and whole grains, women can fortify their immune defenses and reduce the risk of falling ill.

Women who prioritize their nutrition benefit from a decreased risk of chronic diseases. A diet rich in fruits, vegetables, whole grains, and lean proteins can help prevent conditions such as heart disease, diabetes, and certain types of cancer. By making informed food choices and adopting a well-balanced eating pattern, women can significantly reduce their risk of developing these life-threatening conditions.

In conclusion, women's nutrition is of paramount importance for overall well-being. By providing the body with nutrients, women can enjoy increased energy levels, a strengthened immune system, and a reduced risk of chronic diseases. Prioritizing nutrition allows women to nourish their bodies and minds, enabling them to lead healthy, fulfilling lives.

THE UNIQUE NUTRITIONAL NEEDS OF WOMEN

As women, our bodies go through various stages and experiences that significantly affect our nutritional needs. Whether it's puberty, pregnancy, menopause, or the general demands of a busy lifestyle, understanding and addressing our unique nutritional needs is essential for optimal health and well-being.

Puberty is the stage where our bodies undergo significant hormonal changes, leading to the development of secondary sexual characteristics. During this time, proper nutrition becomes crucial to support our growth and development. Adequate intake of calcium, iron, and vitamin D is essential to ensure healthy bone development and prevent issues like osteoporosis later in life. Consuming a balanced diet rich in fruits, vegetables, whole grains, and lean proteins helps maintain a healthy weight and promotes overall well-being.

Pregnancy is another phase in a woman's life that requires special attention to nutrition. During this time, the body needs extra nutrients to support the growth and development of the baby. Folic acid, iron, calcium, and omega-3 fatty acids are important during pregnancy. These nutrients aid in the baby's formation's neural tube, prevent anemia, support bone health, and contribute to the baby's brain development. It's crucial to consult with a healthcare professional to ensure proper supplementation and dietary choices during pregnancy.

Menopause, the stage when menstruation ceases, brings its own set of challenges. Hormonal changes during menopause can lead to various symptoms such as hot flashes, mood swings, and weight gain. Proper nutrition can help ease these symptoms and support overall health. Increasing the intake of calcium and vitamin D can help maintain bone health, while consuming foods rich in phytoestrogen, such as soy, can help balance hormone levels. A diet high in fruits, vegetables, and whole grains can help manage weight and reduce the risk of chronic diseases.

Overall, women need to focus on maintaining a balanced and varied diet that includes plenty of fruits, vegetables, whole grains, lean proteins, and healthy fats. Regular physical activity is also crucial for maintaining a healthy weight, managing stress, and promoting overall well-being. It's important to remember that each woman's nutritional needs may vary depending on her age, ac

tivity level, and specific health conditions. Consulting with a registered dietitian or healthcare professional can provide personalized guidance to meet individual nutritional needs.

By prioritizing our unique nutritional needs and making conscious choices, women can nourish their bodies and minds, ensuring optimal health and vitality throughout their lives.

CHAPTER 2: BUILDING A HEALTHY FOUNDATION

Establishing Balanced Eating Habits

In today's fast-paced world, it's easy for women to neglect their nutritional needs. Juggling work, family, and personal commitments often leaves little time for proper meal planning and healthy eating. However, prioritizing your nutrition is essential for maintaining optimal health and well-being. This subchapter aims to guide women toward establishing balanced eating habits that nourish both their bodies and minds.

The concept of balanced eating revolves around consuming a variety of nutrient-dense foods in portions. It involves finding the right balance between macronutrients (carbohydrates, proteins, and fats) and micronutrients

(vitamins and minerals) to meet your specific needs. A balanced diet supports overall health, boosts energy levels, promotes mental clarity, and helps manage weight effectively.

One of the key principles of establishing balanced eating habits is to focus on whole, unprocessed foods. Incorporating whole, unprocessed foods into your diet ensures you consume a wide range of nutrients, including plenty of fruits, vegetables, whole grains, lean proteins, and healthy fats. These foods are rich in vitamins, minerals, antioxidants, and fiber, which aid in digestion and prevent chronic diseases.

Another important aspect of balanced eating is portion control. Being mindful of how much you eat helps prevent overeating and promotes a healthy weight. Paying attention to hunger and fullness cues, using smaller plates, and practicing mindful eating can all contribute to portion control.

Hydration plays a vital role in maintaining a balanced diet. Drinking an adequate amount of water throughout the day is crucial for digestion, nutrient absorption, and overall bodily functions. I highly recommended it to limit the intake of sugary beverages and opt for water or herbal teas.

Establishing balanced eating habits also involves being mindful of emotional eating triggers. Women often turn to food for comfort, stress relief, or reward. Recognizing these triggers and finding alternative ways to cope with emotions, such as exercise, meditation, or engaging in hobbies, can help break unhealthy eating patterns.

Finally, seeking professional guidance is essential when establishing balanced eating habits. Consulting a registered dietitian or nutritionist who specializes in women's health can provide personalized advice, address specific dietary concerns, and create a tailored meal plan.

In conclusion, establishing balanced eating habits is crucial for women's overall well-being. By focusing on whole, unprocessed foods, practicing portion control, staying hydrated, being mindful of emotional eating triggers, and seeking professional guidance, women can nourish their bodies and minds, leading to optimal health and vitality.

UNDERSTANDING MACRONUTRIENTS AND MICRONUTRIENTS

To achieve optimal health and nourish your body and mind, it is essential to have a thorough understanding of macronutrients and micronutrients. These two categories of nutrients play a vital role in women's nutrition and healthy eating.

Macronutrients are the nutrients that our bodies require in large quantities to provide energy and support overall bodily functions. The three main macronutrients are carbohydrates, proteins, and fats. Foods like grains, fruits, and vegetables contain carbohydrates, which are the body's major source of energy. Proteins are essential for building and repairing tissues, and we can find them in foods like lean meats, poultry, fish, beans, and legumes. Healthy fats, such as those found in avocados,

nuts, and seeds, are crucial for hormone production and brain function.

The nutrients that our bodies require in smaller quantities are called micronutrients, and they are essential for optimal health. Micronutrients include vitamins and minerals, which are essential for various bodily functions, such as immune system support, bone health, and energy production. We can get vitamins from a variety of sources, including fruits, vegetables, and whole grains. Foods like dairy products, lean meats, and leafy green vegetables contain minerals such as calcium, iron, and zinc.

For women, understanding the importance of macronutrients and micronutrients is crucial for maintaining overall health and well-being. Adequate intake of macronutrients is essential for energy levels, supporting physical activity, and maintaining a healthy weight. Consuming a variety of micronutrients is necessary to support reproductive health, and hormonal balance, and to prevent deficiencies that can lead to various health issues.

To ensure you are getting the right balance of macronutrients and micronutrients, it is important to focus on a well-rounded diet that includes a variety of whole, unprocessed foods. By incorporating a range of fruits, vegetables, whole grains, lean proteins, and healthy fats

into your meals, you can provide your body with the nutrients it needs to function optimally.

In conclusion, understanding macronutrients and micronutrients is essential for women's nutrition and healthy eating. By incorporating a balanced diet that includes a variety of foods rich in macronutrients and micronutrients, women can nourish their bodies and minds, promoting overall health and well-being. Remember, a well-nourished body is a key component of leading a vibrant and fulfilling life.

PORTION CONTROL AND MINDFUL EATING

In today's fast-paced world, it's easy to overlook the importance of portion control and mindful eating. As women, we often juggle multiple responsibilities, leaving little time to focus on our health and nutrition. However, understanding the significance of portion control and practicing mindful eating can have a profound impact on our overall well-being.

Portion control refers to the practice of consuming the amount of food for our bodies' needs. It is vital for maintaining a healthy weight, preventing overeating, and promoting optimal nutrition. Many of us are guilty of mindlessly eating oversized portions, whether because of societal norms, emotional eating, or simply not paying attention. By practicing portion control, we can regain control over our eating habits and nourish our bodies most beneficially.

Mindful eating involves being fully present and aware of our eating experience. It means savoring each bite, paying attention to our body's hunger and fullness cues, and appreciating the flavors and textures of our food. Mindful eating helps us develop a healthier relationship with food and prevents us from eating out of boredom, stress, or habit. By becoming more mindful, we can make conscious choices about what we eat and how much we consume, leading to improved digestion, increased satisfaction, and overall better health.

To practice portion control and mindful eating, there are several strategies we can implement in our daily lives. Foremost, it is essential to listen to our bodies and eat when we are truly hungry, rather than relying on external cues or emotional triggers. Using smaller plates, bowls, and utensils can help control portion sizes and give the illusion of a more substantial meal. Planning and preparing meals in advance, using food scales and measuring cups, and being mindful of serving sizes shown on food labels are also effective ways to manage portion control.

Practicing mindful eating involves eliminating distractions during meals, such as television or scrolling through our phones, and instead focusing on the sensory experience of eating. Chewing slowly, taking small bites, and pausing between each mouthful can help us tune in to our body's signals of fullness and prevent overeating. It is also beneficial to cultivate gratitude for the food we

consume and appreciate the effort that goes into its production, further enhancing our mindful eating practice.

In conclusion, portion control and mindful eating are crucial aspects of optimal nutrition for women. By implementing these practices, we can nourish our bodies and minds, maintain a healthy weight, and develop a positive relationship with food. Let us prioritize our well-being by embracing portion control and mindful eating, one mindful bite at a time.

CHAPTER 3: KEY NUTRIENTS FOR WOMEN'S HEALTH

Calcium and Bone Health

As women, we often hear about the importance of calcium in our bone health, but do we truly understand why it is so crucial? In this subchapter, we will delve into the relationship between calcium and bone health, and explore how we can nourish our bodies to optimize our bone strength.

Calcium is a mineral that plays a vital role in maintaining healthy bones and teeth. Our bodies continuously break down and rebuild bone tissue, and calcium is required for this process. If we don't consume enough calcium, our bones can become weak and brittle, making us more susceptible to fractures and osteoporosis, a condition characterized by low bone density.

Women need to prioritize calcium intake, as we have a higher risk of developing osteoporosis compared to men. This risk is further increased during menopause when estrogen levels decline, as estrogen helps protect our bones. By ensuring we get adequate calcium throughout our lives, we can help minimize the risk of osteoporosis and maintain strong, healthy bones.

So, how much calcium do we need? The recommended daily intake for women aged 19 to 50 is 1000 milligrams, while women over 50 should aim for 1200 milligrams. It's important to note that our bodies can only absorb a certain amount of calcium at a time, so it's best to spread our intake throughout the day rather than consuming it all at once.

While dairy products like milk, yogurt, and cheese are often associated with calcium, there are other excellent sources for those who may be lactose intolerant or prefer non-dairy options. Leafy greens like kale and broccoli, as well as tofu, almonds, and fortified plant-based milk, are all significant sources of calcium.

Besides calcium, it's important to remember that other nutrients play a role in maintaining bone health. Vitamin D, for example, helps our bodies absorb calcium. Spending time in the sun and consuming foods like fatty fish,

fortified cereals, and egg yolks can help ensure we get enough vitamin D.

In conclusion, calcium is a vital mineral for women's bone health. By incorporating calcium-rich foods into our diets and ensuring we meet the recommended daily intake, we can protect our bones and reduce the risk of osteoporosis. Also, consider other nutrients, including vitamin D, that collaborate with calcium to improve bone health to the fullest. Let's nourish our bodies and minds to lead healthier, stronger lives.

Iron and Anemia Prevention

One of the most important aspects of a woman's nutrition is ensuring an adequate intake of iron. Iron is an essential mineral that plays a vital role in the body, particularly in the production of red blood cells. Unfortunately, many women suffer from iron deficiency, which can lead to a condition called anemia. This subchapter will explore the significance of iron in women's nutrition and provide valuable insights into preventing anemia.

Iron is crucial for the transportation of oxygen throughout the body. It is a key component of hemoglobin, a protein found in red blood cells that carries oxygen from the lungs to all tissues and organs. Without sufficient iron, the body cannot produce enough healthy red blood cells,

leading to anemia. Anemia can cause fatigue, weakness, pale skin, and difficulty concentrating, among other symptoms. It can significantly affect a woman's overall well-being and quality of life.

To prevent anemia, women need to consume iron-rich foods regularly. There are two types of dietary iron: heme and non-heme iron. We find heme iron in animal sources such as red meat, poultry, and seafood, and is more easily absorbed by the body. Plant-based sources like beans, lentils, spinach, and fortified cereals contain non-heme iron.

While animal sources of iron are often more readily absorbed, it is still possible for women to follow vegetarian or vegan diets to meet their iron needs. To enhance the absorption of non-heme iron, we recommend it to consume these foods with vitamin C-rich foods like citrus fruits, tomatoes, or bell peppers, as vitamin C aids in iron absorption.

Certain factors can hinder iron absorption. For instance, calcium and tannins found in tea and coffee can inhibit iron absorption, so it is advisable to consume these beverages separately from iron-rich meals. Women experiencing heavy menstrual bleeding or pregnant women may require additional iron supplementation, as their iron needs are higher.

In conclusion, iron plays a crucial role in women's nutrition, and its deficiency can lead to anemia. By incorporating iron-rich foods into their diets and paying attention to factors that can hinder iron absorption, women can take steps to prevent anemia and maintain optimal health.

FOLATE AND PREGNANCY

One of the most crucial nutrients for women during pregnancy is folate. Also known as vitamin B9, folate plays a vital role in the development of a healthy baby and can prevent certain birth defects. This subchapter will explore the importance of folate during pregnancy and provide practical tips on how to incorporate it into your diet.

During pregnancy, folate is essential for the growth and division of cells, especially during the early stages of fetal development. It helps in the formation of the neural tube, which later develops into the baby's brain and spinal cord. Adequate folate intake is crucial in reducing the risk of neural tube defects, such as spina bifida and anencephaly.

To ensure optimal folate levels, we recommend that women who are planning to conceive or are in the early stages of pregnancy consume at least 400 to 800 micro

grams (mcg) of folate daily. We can achieve this through a combination of folate-rich foods and supplements.

Leafy green vegetables such as spinach, kale, and broccoli are excellent sources of folate. Other foods rich in this nutrient include citrus fruits, legumes, nuts, and whole grains. Incorporating these foods into your daily meals can help you meet your folate requirements naturally. Experts recommend consuming some raw or lightly cooked foods, as cooking and processing methods can decrease folate levels.

Besides a healthy diet, it commonly recommended prenatal supplements containing folic acid for pregnant women. The body easily absorbed folic acid, which is the synthetic form of folate. It is important to take these supplements even before conception to ensure sufficient folate levels during the early stages of pregnancy.

While folate is essential, it is equally important to avoid excessive intake. High levels of folate can mask a vitamin B12 deficiency, which can have adverse effects on both the mother and baby. Therefore, it is advisable to consult with a healthcare professional or a registered dietitian to determine the dosage for your specific needs.

In conclusion, folate is a vital nutrient for pregnant women, playing a crucial role in the healthy develop

ment of the baby. By incorporating folate-rich foods into your diet and considering folic acid supplements, you can ensure optimal folate levels, reducing the risk of birth defects and promoting a healthy pregnancy. Remember to consult with a healthcare professional for personalized advice on folate intake during this important time.

OMEGA-3 FATTY ACIDS AND HEART HEALTH

Heart disease is a leading cause of death among women worldwide. As women, we must prioritize our heart health and take steps to prevent cardiovascular problems. One powerful tool in our arsenal is the inclusion of omega-3 fatty acids in our diets.

Scientists have extensively studied omega-3 fatty acids, particularly for their positive impact on heart health and many health benefits. These essential fats play a crucial role in reducing inflammation, lowering blood pressure, and decreasing the risk of heart disease.

Research has shown that omega-3 fatty acids can lower triglyceride levels, a type of fat in the blood that can contribute to the development of heart disease. By reducing triglyceride levels, omega-3s help to improve over

all heart health and reduce the risk of heart attacks and strokes.

Researchers have found that omega-3 fatty acids directly reduce the risk of arrhythmias, which are irregular heartbeats that can be life-threatening. By promoting regular heart rhythm, omega-3s contribute to a healthy cardiovascular system.

Besides their cardiovascular benefits, omega-3 fatty acids also play a crucial role in brain health. They are essential for the development and functioning of the brain and can help improve cognitive function, memory, and mood. As women, we often face unique challenges related to hormonal changes and stress, making omega-3s even more valuable for our overall well-being.

To incorporate more omega-3 fatty acids into your diet, consider adding fatty fish such as salmon, mackerel, and sardines to your meals. You can enjoy these fish grilled, baked, or even canned fish. They are excellent sources of omega-3s.

If you are not a fan of fish, you can also get omega-3 fatty acids from plant sources such as flaxseeds, chia seeds, and walnuts. These vegetarian options offer a great alternative for those following a plant-based diet.

To ensure you are getting enough omega-3s, consider incorporating a high-quality fish oil or algae-based supplement into your daily routine. These supplements are a convenient and reliable way to meet your omega-3 requirements.

Remember, taking care of your heart's health is essential for overall well-being. By including omega-3 fatty acids in your diet, you can nourish your body and mind while reducing the risk of heart disease and promoting optimal health.

VITAMIN D AND IMMUNE SYSTEM SUPPORT

In today's fast-paced world, women often juggle multiple roles and responsibilities. With so much on their plate, it becomes crucial for women to prioritize their health and well-being. One key aspect of maintaining optimal health is nourishing the body and mind through proper nutrition. In this subchapter, we will delve into the fascinating connection between Vitamin D and immune system support, specifically addressing the needs of women.

Vitamin D, often referred to as the "sunshine vitamin," plays a vital role in supporting our immune system. It is a unique nutrient that not only acts as a vitamin but also functions as a hormone within our bodies. While sunlight is the primary source of Vitamin D, we can also get it through certain foods and supplements.

Research has shown that Vitamin D deficiency is prevalent among women, especially those living in regions with limited sunlight exposure or those who follow a strict vegetarian or vegan diet.

This deficiency can lead to a weakened immune system, making women more susceptible to various illnesses and diseases.

A robust immune system is essential for women of all ages, as it helps ward off infections, reduces the risk of chronic diseases, and supports overall well-being. Vitamin D plays a crucial role in this process by regulating and enhancing the function of immune cells. It aids in the production of antimicrobial peptides, which help fight off harmful bacteria, viruses, and fungi.

We have linked vitamin D to reducing the risk of autoimmune diseases such as multiple sclerosis, rheumatoid arthritis, and even certain types of cancers. It also plays a role in preventing respiratory infections, making it even more critical during flu seasons or pandemics.

To ensure optimal immune system support, women need to incorporate Vitamin D-rich foods into their diet. Fatty fish like salmon and mackerel, egg yolks, mushrooms, and fortified dairy products are excellent sources of this essential nutrient. However, it's challenging to get sufficient Vitamin D through diet alone, especially for women with limited sun exposure.

Therefore, it is advisable to consult with a healthcare professional who may recommend Vitamin D supplements based on individual needs and circumstances. Regular blood tests can also help determine if you are deficient in Vitamin D and require supplementation.

In conclusion, Vitamin D plays a crucial role in supporting the immune system of women. By ensuring sufficient intake through a combination of sunlight exposure, dietary sources, and supplements, women can enhance their immune response, reduce the risk of illnesses, and maintain optimal health. Prioritizing Vitamin D as part of a well-rounded nutrition plan is a step towards nourishing not just the body but also the mind, enabling women to thrive in all aspects of their lives.

CHAPTER 4: EATING FOR HORMONAL BALANCE

Understanding Female Hormones

As women, our bodies go through many hormonal changes throughout our lives. From puberty to pregnancy and menopause, hormones play a vital role in our overall health and well-being. Understanding female hormones is essential for maintaining optimal nutrition and promoting healthy eating habits.

One of the most prominent female hormones is estrogen. Estrogen regulates our menstrual cycles and plays a crucial role in reproductive health. It also contributes to the development of secondary sexual characteristics and helps maintain healthy bones and skin. However, an imbalance in estrogen levels can lead to various health issues, including weight gain, mood swings, and even certain types of cancer.

Another vital hormone is progesterone. Progesterone works hand in hand with estrogen to regulate menstrual cycles and support pregnancy. It helps prepare the uterus for implantation and maintains a healthy pregnancy. Low levels of progesterone can cause irregular periods, fertility issues, and difficulty conceiving.

Testosterone, often associated with men, is also present in women, although in smaller amounts. Testosterone plays a role in maintaining muscle mass, bone density, and libido. Imbalances in testosterone levels can lead to decreased sex drive, mood changes, and even hair loss.

Understanding how these hormones interact with each other and impact our overall health allows us to make informed choices about our nutrition and eating habits. A well-balanced diet rich in nutrients can help regulate hormone levels and promote hormonal balance.

Certain foods can support hormone production and balance. For example, foods rich in omega-3 fatty acids, such as salmon and chia seeds, can help regulate estrogen levels. Leafy greens like kale and spinach provide essential nutrients that support progesterone production. Incorporating lean proteins like chicken and tofu can help maintain testosterone levels.

It's also important to be mindful of lifestyle factors that can influence hormonal balance. Regular exercise, stress management techniques like yoga or meditation, and sufficient sleep all contribute to hormonal health.

By understanding how female hormones work and how our nutrition and lifestyle choices can affect them, we can empower ourselves to make informed decisions about our health. With the right knowledge and a balanced approach to nutrition and healthy eating, we can nourish our bodies and minds, supporting optimal hormonal balance and overall well-being.

FOODS TO SUPPORT HORMONAL HEALTH

As women, our bodies go through various hormonal changes throughout our lives. From puberty to pregnancy, and eventually menopause, hormones play a crucial role in our overall health and well-being. One of the most effective ways to support hormonal health is through a balanced and nutritious diet. By incorporating specific foods into our daily meals, we can nourish our bodies and promote hormonal balance.

1. Omega-3 Fatty Acids: These healthy fats found in fatty fish like salmon, sardines, and mackerel, as well as flaxseeds and walnuts, are essential for hormone production and regulation. Omega-3s help reduce inflammation and support brain health, which can ease symptoms of hor

monal imbalances such as mood swings and irregular periods.

2. Cruciferous Vegetables: broccoli, cauliflower, kale, and Brussels sprouts are excellent sources of fiber and contain compounds that support the detoxification of excess hormones. These vegetables also contain indole-3-carbinol, which helps balance estrogen levels and reduce the risk of estrogen-related cancers.

3. Fiber-rich Foods: Whole grains, legumes, fruits, and vegetables are high in fiber, which aids in hormonal balance by promoting healthy digestion and eliminating excess hormones from the body. Fiber also helps regulate blood sugar levels, reducing the risk of insulin resistance and supporting balanced hormone production.

4. Healthy Fats: Avocados, olive oil, and nuts are rich in monounsaturated fats that support hormone production and absorption. These fats also provide a steady source of energy and promote satiety, preventing overeating and weight gain, which can disrupt hormonal balance.

5. Fermented Foods: yogurt, kefir, sauerkraut, and kimchi are examples of fermented foods that contain probiotics. Probiotics help balance gut bacteria, which plays a crucial role in hormone metabolism and production. A healthy gut microbiome can ease symptoms of hormonal

imbalances, such as bloating and irregular bowel movements.

6. Adaptogenic Herbs: Adaptogens like mica, ashwagandha, and holy basil helps the body adapt to stress and support hormone regulation. These herbs can help ease symptoms of adrenal fatigue, improve sleep quality, and reduce anxiety, all of which contribute to hormonal health.

Incorporating these foods into your daily diet can support hormonal health and overall well-being. Remember to prioritize whole, unprocessed foods and listen to your body's unique needs. Consult with a healthcare professional or a registered dietitian to create a personalized nutrition plan tailored to your specific hormonal health goals. Nourishing your body with the right foods will not only support hormone balance but also promote optimal nutrition for your body and mind.

MANAGING PMS SYMPTOMS THROUGH NUTRITION

Introduction

As women, we are all too familiar with the discomfort and mood swings that come along with premenstrual syndrome (PMS). However, did you know that the food you eat can play a significant role in managing these symptoms? In this subchapter, we will explore how nutrition can be a powerful tool in alleviating PMS symptoms and improving overall well-being.

Understanding PMS

Premenstrual syndrome is a combination of physical and emotional symptoms that occur in the days leading up to your menstrual period. Symptoms can vary from bloating, fatigue, and headaches to irritability, mood swings, and depression. Although the exact cause of PMS is still unknown, experts believe that hormonal changes, imbalances in neurotransmitters, and nutritional deficiencies contribute to these symptoms.

The Role of Nutrition

A balanced and nutrient-rich diet can help regulate hormones, improve mood, reduce inflammation, and support overall well-being. Here are some dietary tips to help manage PMS symptoms:

1. Increase Complex Carbohydrates:

Including whole grains, legumes, and starchy vegetables in your diet can help stabilize blood sugar levels, reduce cravings, and improve mood swings.

2. Opt for Healthy Fats:

Omega-3 fatty acids found in fatty fish, flaxseeds, and walnuts have anti-inflammatory properties and can help reduce bloating and breast tenderness.

3. Boost Vitamin B Intake:

We have shown vitamin B6 to ease PMS symptoms, including bloating, irritability, and breast pain. Incorporate foods like bananas, spinach, poultry, and whole grains into your diet.

4. Prioritize Calcium and Magnesium:

These minerals are essential for muscle relaxation and mood regulation. Include calcium-rich foods like dairy products, leafy greens, and fortified plant-based milk, along with magnesium-rich foods such as nuts, seeds, and dark chocolate.

5. Reduce Salt and Caffeine Intake:

Both salt and caffeine can contribute to bloating and breast tenderness. Limit your consumption of processed foods, salty snacks, and caffeinated beverages during the premenstrual phase.

Conclusion:

While PMS symptoms can be challenging to deal with, making simple dietary changes can have a significant impact on your overall well-being. By incorporating nutrient-dense foods and avoiding triggers like salt and caffeine, you can effectively manage PMS symptoms and experience a smoother menstrual cycle. Remember, your body deserves the best nourishment, and by taking care of your nutritional needs, you can support a healthier and happier you.

CHAPTER 5: NOURISHING YOUR BODY DURING DIFFERENT LIFE STAGES

Nutrition for Adolescence

During adolescence, young women experience significant physical and emotional changes, making it a crucial period for proper nutrition and healthy eating habits. This subchapter explores the unique nutritional needs of adolescent girls and provides valuable insights into nourishing their bodies and minds.

1. Understanding the Adolescent Growth Spurt:

The adolescent growth spurt is a period characterized by rapid physical growth, bone development, and hormonal changes. Adequate nutrition is essential to support this growth and ensure optimal development. This section discusses the specific nutrients required during this phase, such as calcium, iron, vitamin D, and protein.

2. Balancing Energy Intake:

Adolescent girls often face challenges in balancing their energy intake because of various factors such as increased social activities, academic pressures, and body image concerns. This subchapter addresses the importance of maintaining a balanced diet and provides practical tips to help young women make informed food choices.

3. Promoting Healthy Body Image:

Adolescence is a critical time for body image development, and poor nutrition choices can contribute to negative body image issues. This section emphasizes the importance of fostering a healthy body image and educates young women on the connection between nutrition, self-esteem, and body confidence.

4. Meal Planning and Snacking:

To meet their nutritional needs, adolescent girls should focus on well-rounded meals and incorporate healthy snacks into their daily routines. This subchapter discusses the importance of meal planning, portion control, and mindful eating. It also offers simple and nutritious snack ideas that promote optimal health and energy levels.

5. Navigating Fad Diets and Eating Disorders:

Young women may adopt unhealthy eating habits or fad diets due to societal pressures during adolescence. This section addresses the risks. This section addresses the risks associated with fad diets and guides how to recognize and address potential eating disorders, emphasizing the importance of a balanced and sustainable approach to nutrition.

6. Addressing Nutrient Deficiencies:

Adolescent girls are at a higher risk of developing nutrient deficiencies, such as iron deficiency anemia or calcium insufficiency. This subchapter highlights the importance of regular check-ups and blood tests to identify and address any potential deficiencies. It also provides insights into incorporating nutrient-rich foods into the diet to prevent deficiencies.

In conclusion, adolescence is a crucial phase for young women to establish healthy eating habits that will positively affect their overall well-being. This subchapter equips women with the knowledge and tools necessary to navigate the unique nutritional challenges they face during this transformative period. By nourishing their bodies and minds, adolescent girls can thrive and lay the foundation for a lifetime of optimal nutrition and wellness.

EATING WELL DURING REPRODUCTIVE YEARS

As women, our reproductive years are a special time in our lives. Whether you are planning to conceive, are currently pregnant, or are navigating the challenges of postpartum, it is crucial to prioritize your nutrition and overall well-being. This subchapter aims to guide you on how to eat well during your reproductive years, ensuring that you nourish your body and mind.

During the reproductive years, a balanced and nutrient-rich diet is essential for supporting fertility, a healthy pregnancy, and postpartum recovery. The foods you choose can have a significant impact on your reproductive health and overall vitality.

Foremost, focus on consuming a variety of whole foods. Include plenty of fruits, vegetables, whole grains, lean proteins, and healthy fats in your diet. They packed these foods with essential vitamins, minerals, and antioxidants that support reproductive health.

Incorporate foods rich in folate, such as leafy greens, citrus fruits, and legumes. Folate is crucial for preventing neural tube defects in babies and is especially important during the preconception period. Ensure you are getting enough iron from sources like lean meats, dark leafy greens, and beans to support healthy blood production.

Fatty fish, flaxseeds, and walnuts contain omega-3 fatty acids that are vital for reproductive health. These healthy fats play a role in hormone production, and fetal brain development, and can help ease symptoms of postpartum depression.

Stay hydrated by drinking plenty of water throughout the day. Water is essential for maintaining optimal bodily functions, including digestion, circulation, and hormone balance.

Besides a healthy diet, consider taking quality prenatal vitamins during your reproductive years, especially if you are planning to conceive. Prenatal vitamins provide

essential nutrients like folic acid, iron, and calcium that are crucial for a healthy pregnancy.

Last, prioritize self-care and stress management. Stress can negatively affect reproductive health, so relax and unwind. Engage in activities that bring you joy, practice mindfulness or meditation, and ensure you are getting enough sleep.

Remember, every woman's reproductive journey is unique, so it is essential to listen to your body and work with a healthcare professional or registered dietitian to tailor your nutrition plan to your specific needs.

By nourishing your body with a balanced diet, staying hydrated, and practicing self-care, you can optimize your reproductive health and overall well-being during these special years.

SUPPORTING MENOPAUSE WITH PROPER NUTRITION

Menopause is a natural phase in a woman's life that signifies the end of her reproductive years. While menopause brings about various physical and emotional changes, it is essential to understand that proper nutrition plays a crucial role in supporting women through this transition. By focusing on a well-balanced diet and making mindful food choices, women can ease symptoms and promote overall well-being during this transformative time.

One of the primary concerns during menopause is maintaining healthy bones. As estrogen levels decline, women become more susceptible to bone loss and osteoporosis. To combat this, it is crucial to include calcium-rich foods in your diet. Dairy products, such as milk, cheese, and

yogurt, are excellent sources of calcium. However, if you are lactose intolerant or following a plant-based diet, you can opt for alternatives like fortified plant-based milk, leafy green vegetables, and tofu.

Another important nutrient to include is vitamin D, as it aids in calcium absorption. Sunlight is the primary source of vitamin D, but during menopause, women may need additional supplementation. Fatty fish like salmon, eggs, and fortified cereals are also excellent sources of this essential vitamin.

During menopause, hormonal changes can lead to weight gain and an increased risk of heart disease. To combat these issues, it is essential to focus on a diet that includes whole grains, lean proteins, and healthy fats. Whole grains provide fiber, which aids in digestion and helps manage weight. Opt for whole wheat bread, brown rice, and quinoa. Lean proteins like poultry, fish, and legumes help build and repair tissues while providing a feeling of fullness. Healthy fats, such as those found in avocados, nuts, and olive oil, are beneficial for heart health.

Menopause can bring about mood swings, irritability, and sleep disturbances. Including foods rich in omega-3 fatty acids, such as fatty fish, walnuts, and flaxseeds, can help ease these symptoms. Fatty fish, walnuts, and flaxseeds are foods rich in omega-3 fatty acids. They support brain health and ease mood swings, irritability, and sleep disturbances caused by menopause.

In conclusion, menopause is a natural phase in a woman's life that requires proper nutrition for optimal well-being. By incorporating calcium-rich foods, vitamin D, whole grains, lean proteins, healthy fats, and omega-3 fatty acids, women can support their bodies and minds during this transformative time. Remember to consult with a healthcare professional or registered dietitian to create a personalized nutrition plan that best suits your needs. Embracing a balanced and nutritious diet during menopause will empower women to navigate this phase with grace and vitality.

CHAPTER 6: NUTRITIONAL STRATEGIES FOR OPTIMAL MENTAL HEALTH

The Gut-Brain Connection

The Gut-Brain Connection: Nourishing Your Body and Mind

In recent years, researchers have uncovered the fascinating and intricate relationship between our gut and brain. This connection, known as the gut-brain axis, plays a crucial role in our overall health and well-being. As women, understanding and nurturing this connection can have a profound impact on our nutrition and overall vitality.

The gut-brain connection refers to the constant communication and feedback loop between our gut and the brain. It involves complex interactions between the nervous system, immune system, and gut microbiota, which are the trillions of bacteria that live in our digestive tract. This intricate network influences not only our digestion but also our mood, cognitive function, and even our immune response.

For women, the gut-brain connection is of particular importance because of the unique hormonal fluctuations we experience throughout our lives. Hormonal changes during puberty, pregnancy, and menopause can directly affect the gut microbiota composition, leading to digestive issues, mood swings, and even mental health disorders.

Nurturing this connection starts with a balanced and nourishing diet. Consuming a variety of whole, unprocessed foods such as fruits, vegetables, whole grains, lean proteins, and healthy fats can provide essential nutrients for both our gut and brain. Fiber-rich foods, in particular, support a healthy gut by promoting the growth of beneficial bacteria and aiding in regular bowel movements.

Incorporating fermented foods, such as yogurt, sauerkraut, and kimchi, can introduce beneficial probiotics into our gut, which can positively influence our mood

and cognitive function. They have shown these probiotics to reduce anxiety and depression symptoms and enhance overall mental well-being.

Another essential aspect of nurturing the gut-brain connection is managing stress. Chronic stress can disrupt the balance of gut bacteria and impair digestion. Engaging in stress-reducing activities such as meditation, yoga, or deep breathing exercises can help restore this balance and improve gut health.

Understanding the impact of hormonal changes on our gut health is crucial. During different stages of our lives, we may need to adjust our diet and lifestyle to support hormonal balance and gut health. Consulting with a healthcare professional or registered dietitian who specializes in women's health can provide personalized guidance and support.

By nourishing our gut-brain connection, we empower ourselves to optimize our nutrition and overall well-being as women. Through mindful eating, stress management, and a focus on hormonal balance, we can create a harmonious relationship between our gut and brain, fostering optimal physical and mental health.

FOODS THAT PROMOTE MENTAL WELL-BEING

In today's fast-paced and demanding world, women often juggle many responsibilities and face various challenges that can take a toll on their mental well-being. However, there is a powerful tool right in the hands of every woman that can positively affect her mental health: nutrition. The foods we consume play a crucial role in nourishing both our bodies and minds. In this subchapter, we will explore a range of delicious and nutrient-packed foods that promote mental well-being and help women achieve optimal nutrition.

1. Dark Leafy Greens: Spinach, kale, and Swiss chard are rich in essential vitamins and minerals that support brain health. They are high in folate, which aids in the production of neurotransmitters that regulate mood.

2. Fatty fish like salmon, mackerel, and sardines contain omega-3 fatty acids, which are linked to a reduced risk of depression and anxiety. These healthy fats also support brain function and

enhance cognitive abilities.

3. Berries such as blueberries, strawberries, and blackberries contain antioxidants that shield brain cells against oxidative stress and inflammation. Regular consumption of berries has been associated with improved memory and cognitive function.

4. Whole Grains: Opt for whole grains like quinoa, brown rice, and whole wheat bread to provide your brain with a steady supply of energy. These complex carbohydrates also stimulate the production of serotonin, a neurotransmitter that promotes calmness and happiness.

5. Nuts and seeds: Almonds, walnuts, and flaxseeds are rich in healthy fats, vitamins, and minerals that support brain health. They are also a significant source of protein, which helps stabilize blood sugar levels and maintain a balanced mood.

6. Fermented Foods: Incorporate fermented foods like yogurt, sauerkraut, and kimchi into your diet to support a healthy gut. Research suggests that a healthy gut microbiome positively influences brain function and mood.

7. Dark Chocolate: Indulge in a small piece of dark chocolate, which contains antioxidants and stimulates the release of endorphins, promoting feelings of pleasure and relaxation.

Remember, a well-nourished body leads to a well-nourished mind. By incorporating these foods into your daily diet, you can take steps toward promoting your mental well-being. Embrace the power of nutrition and make choices that fuel both your body and mind, allowing you to thrive in all aspects of life.

MANAGING STRESS THROUGH NUTRITION

Introduction:

In today's fast-paced world, women often juggle multiple responsibilities, leaving little time for self-care and relaxation. As stress levels rise, it becomes crucial to find effective ways to manage it. While there is no magic solution, one powerful tool in your arsenal is nutrition. The food you eat plays a vital role in your overall well-being, including your ability to handle stress. You can manage stress effectively by ensuring that they nourish your body and mind through proper nutrition.

1. Understanding the Connection:

Stress can take a toll on your body, leading to an increased risk of various health issues. This is where nutrition comes into play. By providing your body with the right nutrients, you can build resilience and better cope with stress. They have shown certain foods and nutrients to have a calming effect on the body, while others can exacerbate stress levels.

2. Mindful Eating:

One effective way to manage stress through nutrition is by practicing mindful eating. This involves being fully present in the moment while eating, paying attention to the taste, texture, and smell of the food. By slowing down and savoring each bite, you can enhance the digestive process and promote a sense of calm.

3. Stress-Busting Nutrients:

We have found certain nutrients to have a positive impact on stress levels. For example, foods rich in omega-3 fatty acids, such as salmon and walnuts, can help reduce anxiety and depression. Incorporating magnesium-rich foods like leafy greens, nuts, and whole grains can help regulate stress hormones. Including vitamin C-rich foods, such as citrus fruits and bell peppers, can also support your body's ability to handle stress.

4. The Gut-Brain Connection:

Did you know that there is a strong connection between your gut and brain? The gut microbiome plays a crucial role in regulating mood and stress levels. Including probiotic-rich foods like yogurt and fermented vegetables in your diet can support a healthy gut and positively affect your mental well-being.

5. Avoiding Stress Aggravators:

While some foods can help manage stress, others can worsen it. It's important to be aware of stress aggravators like caffeine, refined sugars, and processed foods. These can cause energy crashes, mood swings, and inflammation, making it harder for your body to handle stress effectively.

Conclusion:

Managing stress through nutrition is a powerful approach to nurturing your body and mind. By adopting mindful eating practices and incorporating stress-busting nutrients, you can build resilience and better cope with the demands of daily life. Remember, nourishing your body with the right foods not only helps manage stress but also promotes overall health and well-being. So, start making conscious choices and prioritize your nutrition to thrive in a stress-filled world.

CHAPTER 7: MAINTAINING A HEALTHY WEIGHT

Understanding Energy Balance

In the journey towards optimal nutrition and overall well-being, one concept that holds paramount importance is energy balance. As women, we lead diverse lives, often juggling multiple responsibilities, and it becomes essential to nurture our bodies and minds with the right nutrition. This subchapter aims to delve into the intricacies of energy balance, shedding light on its significance and providing practical insights into nutrition and healthy eating for women.

Energy balance refers to the equilibrium between the energy we consume through food and beverages and the energy we spend through physical activity and bodily functions. Achieving a harmonious energy balance is crucial for maintaining a healthy weight, promoting

vitality, and preventing chronic diseases. By understanding the dynamics of energy balance, we can make informed choices about our diet, ensuring that our bodies receive the nourishment they need.

To comprehend energy balance, we must first examine two fundamental components: energy intake and energy expenditure. Energy intake represents the calories we consume from the foods we eat and the liquids we drink. Energy expenditure encompasses the calories we burn through physical activity, digestion, and basic bodily functions, such as breathing and regulating body temperature.

As women, our energy needs vary based on factors such as age, body composition, activity level, and reproductive stage. It is essential to balance energy intake and expenditure to maintain a healthy weight and support optimal functioning. Consuming nutrient-dense foods, such as whole grains, lean proteins, colorful fruits and vegetables, and healthy fats, can provide energy while nourishing our bodies.

Understanding portion sizes, listening to our body's hunger and satiety cues, and developing a mindful eating practice can aid in achieving energy balance. Engaging in regular physical activity, whether through structured exercise or simple lifestyle modifications, helps spend energy and boosts overall well-being.

By grasping the concept of energy balance, we empower ourselves to make conscious choices about our nutrition and lifestyle. This knowledge enables us to fuel our bodies with the right nutrients, manage our weight effectively, and promote long-term health and vitality.

In the subsequent chapters, we will delve deeper into specific nutrients, meal planning strategies, and lifestyle habits that can further enhance our understanding of energy balance and guide us toward optimal nutrition, enabling us to nourish both our bodies and minds.

STRATEGIES FOR HEALTHY WEIGHT LOSS

Achieving and maintaining a healthy weight is a common concern among women. In today's fast-paced world, it is essential to adopt effective strategies that promote sustainable weight loss and overall well-being. This subchapter aims to provide women with practical strategies for healthy weight loss, focusing on nutrition and healthy eating habits.

1. Set Realistic Goals:

Start by setting realistic weight loss goals. Remember, healthy weight loss is gradual and sustainable. Aim for losing 1-2 pounds per week, as this allows your body to adjust and prevents drastic weight fluctuations.

2. Embrace Balanced Nutrition:

Adopting a balanced diet is crucial for healthy weight loss. Focus on consuming whole foods such as fruits, vegetables, whole grains, lean proteins, and healthy fats. Avoid processed foods, sugary snacks, and drinks high in calories. Incorporate nutrient-dense foods to support your body's needs.

3. Mindful Eating:

Practicing mindful eating is a powerful strategy for weight loss. Pay attention to your body's hunger and fullness cues. Slow down during meals, savor each bite, and listen to your body's signals of satisfaction. This helps prevent overeating and promotes a healthier relationship with food.

4. Portion Control:

Learning portion control is key to managing calorie intake. Use smaller plates and bowls to control portion sizes visually. Be mindful of portion sizes when eating out or ordering takeout. Aim to fill half your plate with vegetables, one-quarter with lean protein, and one-quarter with whole grains.

5. Regular Meal Patterns:

Establishing regular meal patterns helps regulate blood sugar levels and prevents overeating. Aim to eat three balanced meals and two small snacks evenly spaced throughout the day. Avoid skipping meals or restricting calories, as this can lead to unhealthy eating patterns and slower metabolism.

6. Stay Hydrated:

Proper hydration is often overlooked, but crucial for weight loss. Drinking enough water helps control appetite, aids digestion, and boosts metabolism. Aim to drink at least 8 cups (64 ounces) of water daily and replace sugary beverages with herbal tea or infused water for added flavor.

7. Physical Activity:

Incorporating regular physical activity into your routine speeds up weight loss and improves overall health. Engage in activities you enjoy, such as walking, jogging, swimming, or dancing. Aim for at least 150 minutes of moderate-intensity exercise or 75 minutes of vigorous exercise each week.

Conclusion:

Adopting these strategies for healthy weight loss will not only help you achieve your desired weight but also promote overall well-being. Remember, maintaining a healthy weight is a lifelong journey, and it is essential to create sustainable habits rather than resorting to quick fixes. By nourishing your body with balanced nutrition, practicing mindful eating, and incorporating regular physical activity, you can achieve optimal weight and embrace a healthier lifestyle.

BUILDING A SUSTAINABLE EXERCISE ROUTINE

In today's fast-paced world, it can be challenging for women to find the time and motivation to prioritize exercise. However, building a sustainable exercise routine is crucial for maintaining optimal health and overall well-being. Regular physical activity not only helps in managing weight, but also reduces the risk of chronic diseases, improves mental health, and boosts energy levels. This subchapter will guide women on how to create a sustainable exercise routine that fits their lifestyle, focusing on nutrition and healthy eating for women.

1. Set realistic goals: Start by setting achievable goals that align with your fitness level and lifestyle. Whether it's losing weight, improving cardiovascular endurance, or building strength, having specific goals will help you stay motivated and measure your progress.

2. Find activities you enjoy: Experiment with different exercises to discover what you genuinely enjoy. Whether it's swimming, dancing, yoga, or weightlifting, incorporating activities you love

will make it easier to stick to your routine.

3. Create a schedule: Plan your exercise routine by setting aside dedicated time slots for physical activity. Treat these sessions as important appointments and prioritize them in your daily schedule.

4. Mix it up: Avoid getting stuck in a workout rut by incorporating a variety of exercises. This not only prevents boredom but also challenges different muscle groups, leading to a more balanced and effective routine.

5. Focus on nutrition: Fueling your body with the right nutrients is essential for supporting your exercise routine. Prioritize a well-balanced diet that includes lean proteins, whole grains, fruits, vegetables, and healthy fats. Hydration is also crucial, so drink plenty of water throughout the day.

6. Listen to your body: Pay attention to your body's signals and adjust your routine accordingly. Rest days are just as crucial as exercise days, allowing your body to recover and prevent overstraining. If you experience pain

or discomfort, consult a healthcare professional for guidance.

7. Make it a habit: Consistency is key to building a sustainable exercise routine. Aim for at least 150 minutes of moderate-intensity aerobic activity or 75 minutes of vigorous-intensity activity per week, along with strength training exercises twice a week. Start with small steps and accumulate the duration and intensity of your workouts.

By following these guidelines, women can create a sustainable exercise routine that fits their lifestyle and promotes optimal nutrition and healthy eating. Remember, the journey towards a healthier and fitter begin with taking that first step toward building a sustainable exercise routine.

CHAPTER 8: OVERCOMING COMMON NUTRITIONAL CHALLENGES

Emotional Eating and Food Cravings

For many women, food is not just a source of nourishment; it can also be a way to cope with emotions. Whether it's stress, sadness, boredom, or even happiness, it's common to turn to food for comfort. We know this phenomenon as emotional eating, and it can have a significant impact on both our physical and mental well-being.

Emotional eating and food cravings often go hand in hand. When we experience intense emotions, particu

larly negative ones, our bodies naturally crave foods that provide instant pleasure or temporary relief. These foods are typically high in sugar, fat, or salt, triggering the release of feel-good chemicals in our brains. However, the satisfaction gained from indulging in these cravings is short-lived, leaving us feeling guilty, bloated, and unsatisfied in the long run.

Understanding the triggers for emotional eating is crucial to breaking this cycle. Stress, for instance, can lead to a cascade of hormonal changes in our bodies, which can increase our appetite and make us more prone to reaching for unhealthy foods. Identifying these triggers and finding alternative ways to cope with emotions is key to overcoming emotional eating.

In "The Women's Guide to Optimal Nutrition: Nourishing Your Body and Mind," we dive deep into this topic and offer practical strategies to help you regain control over your relationship with food. We explore various techniques, such as mindfulness, journaling, and stress management, to address the root causes of emotional eating. By becoming more aware of our emotions and learning healthier ways to manage them, we can break free from the cycle of emotional eating.

The book emphasizes the importance of nourishing our bodies with wholesome, nutrient-dense foods. We pro

vide a comprehensive guide to optimal nutrition for women, focusing on the unique dietary needs and challenges faced by women at different stages of life. By adopting a balanced and mindful approach to eating, we can fuel our bodies with the nutrients they need while also enjoying the pleasure of food.

"The Women's Guide to Optimal Nutrition: Nourishing Your Body and Mind" is an empowering resource for women who want to develop a healthy relationship with food, overcome emotional eating, and prioritize their overall well-being. It offers practical advice, expert insights, and real-life stories to inspire and guide women on their journey toward optimal nutrition and a balanced mind-body connection.

Remember, you have the power to nourish your body and mind. Let this book be your guide to unlocking the potential for a healthier, happier you.

Nutrition for Polycystic Ovary Syndrome (PCOS)

Polycystic Ovary Syndrome (PCOS) is a common hormonal disorder that affects many women of reproductive age. The formation of cysts characterizes the ovaries, irregular menstrual cycles, and hormonal imbalances. While the exact cause of PCOS is still unknown, research suggests that nutrition and lifestyle factors play a significant role in managing the symptoms and improving overall health.

For nutrition for PCOS, the focus should be on maintaining a balanced diet that supports hormonal balance, manages insulin resistance, and promotes weight management. Here are some key dietary considerations for women with PCOS:

1. Focus on whole, nutrient-dense foods: opt for fresh fruits, vegetables, whole grains, lean proteins, and healthy fats. These foods provide essential vitamins, minerals, and fiber while keeping you satiated.

2. Control carbohydrate intake: PCOS is often associated with insulin resistance, which can lead to weight gain and difficulty in managing blood sugar levels. Limiting refined carbohydrates, such as white bread, pasta, and sugary snacks, can help stabilize insulin levels and manage weight.

3. Make sure to include lean sources of protein like poultry, fish, tofu, and legumes in every meal. Protein helps regulate blood sugar levels, promotes satiety, and supports muscle growth and repair.

4. Choose healthy fats: Include sources of healthy fats, such as avocados, nuts, seeds, and olive oil, in your diet. These fats help balance hormones and promote overall wellbeing.

5. Be mindful of portion sizes: While it's important to include a variety of nutritious foods in your diet, portion control is key. Pay attention to your body's hunger and fullness cues to avoid overeating.

6. Stay hydrated: Drinking an adequate amount of water is essential for overall health. Aim for at least 8 glasses of water per day to stay hydrated and support proper bodily functions.

7. Consider supplements: In some cases, supplementation may be necessary to address specific nutrient deficiencies associated with PCOS. Consult with a healthcare professional to determine if you need any additional supplements.

Remember, managing PCOS through nutrition is a lifelong commitment. Changing your diet and embracing a healthy lifestyle can have a positive impact on your symptoms and overall wellbeing. Regular exercise, stress management, and sufficient sleep are also crucial components of managing PCOS. Consult with a registered dietitian or healthcare professional to create a personalized nutrition plan that suits your individual needs.

MANAGING MENSTRUAL IRREGULARITIES THROUGH DIET

For women's health, menstrual irregularities can often be a cause of concern and discomfort. From heavy or prolonged periods to painful cramps and hormonal imbalances, these issues can significantly affect a woman's overall well-being. While various factors contribute to these irregularities, diet plays a crucial role in managing and easing these symptoms. In this subchapter, we will explore how proper nutrition and healthy eating habits can help women maintain optimal menstrual health.

One of the key aspects of managing menstrual irregularities through diet is maintaining a balanced intake of essential nutrients. Iron, for example, is essential for replenishing blood loss during menstruation. Including iron-rich foods such as lean meats, leafy greens, and

legumes in your diet can help prevent iron deficiency anemia and reduce fatigue commonly associated with heavy periods.

Another important nutrient to focus on is calcium. They have linked low calcium levels to an increased risk of premenstrual syndrome (PMS) symptoms such as mood swings and menstrual cramps. Incorporating dairy products, fortified plant-based milk, and leafy greens into your meals can help ensure you are meeting your daily calcium needs.

Research has shown that including foods rich in omega-3 fatty acids like salmon, trout, flaxseeds, and walnuts can reduce inflammation and ease menstrual pain. Including these foods in your diet can help manage discomfort during your period.

Besides these specific nutrients, adopting an overall healthy eating pattern is crucial for managing menstrual irregularities. Consuming a diet rich in fruits, vegetables, whole grains, and lean proteins while limiting processed foods, sugary snacks, and caffeine can help regulate hormone levels and reduce inflammation.

It is also essential to stay well-hydrated throughout your menstrual cycle. Drinking plenty of water can help ease bloating and prevent constipation, common issues during menstruation.

Incorporating stress management techniques such as meditation, yoga, and regular exercise can positively impact menstrual health. They have shown stress to affect hormone levels and exacerbate menstrual symptoms. Engaging in activities that promote relaxation and reduce stress can help restore hormonal balance and ease menstrual irregularities.

By paying attention to your diet and making conscious choices to nourish your body, you can effectively manage menstrual irregularities and promote optimal menstrual health. Prioritizing nutrient-rich foods, maintaining a balanced eating pattern, and implementing stress management techniques will support your overall well-being and enhance your quality of life as a woman.

Remember, it is always important to consult with a healthcare professional for personalized advice and guidance tailored to your specific needs and health conditions.

CHAPTER 9: PRACTICAL TIPS FOR EVERYDAY NUTRITION

Meal Planning and Prep for Busy Women

In today's fast-paced world, women often juggle multiple responsibilities, leaving little time for self-care and proper nutrition. However, prioritizing your health and well-being is crucial, and one effective way to do so is through meal planning and preparation. By taking control of your diet and ensuring you have nutritious meals readily available, you can fuel your body and mind, leading to optimal health and vitality.

Meal planning is an approach to nutrition that involves organizing your meals and snacks in advance. It not only saves time but also helps you make healthier choices, avoiding impulse eating or relying on unhealthy con

venience foods. As a busy woman, investing a small amount of time in meal planning can yield significant benefits.

Start by establishing a weekly or monthly meal plan. Consider your schedule and plan noting days when you have more time to cook and prepare meals versus busier days when quick and easy options are necessary. Make a list of your favorite recipes and include a variety of nutrient-dense foods, such as lean proteins, whole grains, fruits, vegetables, and healthy fats.

Once you have your meal plan, it's time to prep. Spend a few hours each week chopping vegetables, cooking grains, and preparing proteins in advance. This way, you'll have the building blocks for quick and easy meals throughout the week. Portion your meals into individual containers, making it convenient to grab and go.

Investing in timesaving kitchen gadgets can also streamline your meal preparation process. A slow cooker or Instant Pot allows you to throw ingredients together in the morning and come home to a delicious, home-cooked meal. A blender can help you whip up nutrient-packed smoothies in minutes, perfect for busy mornings or post-workout fuel.

Remember to incorporate balanced and nutritious snacks into your meal plan as well. Keep a stash of pre-portioned nuts, seeds, and dried fruits in your bag or desk drawer for a quick pick-me-up. Greek yogurt, hard-boiled eggs, and cut-up vegetables with hummus are also excellent options to have on hand.

By embracing meal planning and prep, you're not only nourishing your body but also setting yourself up for success. With nutritious meals readily available, you'll have more energy, improved mental clarity, and better overall health. Take control of your nutrition, and you'll find that even amid a busy schedule, you can prioritize your well-being.

SMART GROCERY SHOPPING FOR NUTRITIOUS CHOICES

Making smart choices at the grocery store is essential for maintaining a healthy and balanced diet. As women, our nutritional needs are unique and require careful consideration. This subchapter aims to provide practical advice and tips on how to navigate the aisles and make nutritious choices that benefit both our bodies and minds.

1. Create a shopping list: Before heading to the grocery store, take the time to plan your meals for the week and write the ingredients you need. This will help you stay focused and avoid impulsive purchases of unhealthy foods.

2. Shop the perimeter: The perimeter of the grocery store is where you'll find fresh produce, lean meats, and dairy products. Concentrate on filling your cart with whole

Foods from these sections, as they are typically the most nutritious options.

3. Read labels: When purchasing packaged foods, it's crucial to

read the labels carefully. Look for products that are low in added sugars, sodium, and unhealthy fats. Pay attention to the ingredient list, and opt for items with recognizable and natural ingredients.

4. Choose whole grains: Replace refined grains with whole grains like brown rice, quinoa, and whole wheat bread. These are rich in fiber, vitamins, and minerals that promote good digestion and overall health.

5. Include a variety of fruits and vegetables: Aim to include a wide range of colorful fruits and vegetables in your cart. We packed these with essential nutrients and antioxidants that boost your immune system and support optimal health.

6. Opt for lean proteins: Select lean proteins such as skinless chicken, fish, tofu, and legumes. These provide essential amino acids and are lower in saturated fat, making them healthier choices for women.

7. Don't forget healthy fats: Include sources of healthy fats in your shopping list, such as avocados, nuts, seeds,

and olive oil. These fats are beneficial for heart health and help with nutrient absorption.

8. Beware of marketing tactics: Be cautious of marketing claims such as "low-fat" or "sugar-free." These products may still be high in unhealthy additives or artificial sweeteners. Always read the labels and make informed choices.

9. Plan for snacks: Choose wholesome snacks like Greek yogurt,

fresh fruit, or a handful of nuts. By having these options readily available, you'll be less likely to reach for processed and less nutritious alternatives.

10. Stay hydrated: Don't forget to include water in your grocery list. Staying hydrated is crucial for overall health and can help control cravings and overeating.

By following these guidelines, you can make smart grocery shopping choices that empower you to nourish your body and mind. Remember, the key is to be mindful of your nutritional needs and prioritize whole, unprocessed foods for optimal health and well-being.

EATING OUT AND MAKING HEALTHY CHOICES

In today's fast-paced world, eating out has become a regular part of our lives. Whether it's grabbing a quick bite during lunch breaks or indulging in a fancy dinner with friends, dining out can be both convenient and enjoyable. However, it can also pose challenges for women who are conscious of their nutrition and overall health.

In this subchapter, we will explore practical strategies and tips that will empower women to make healthier choices when eating out. By understanding the importance of nutrition and adopting mindful eating habits, women can nourish their bodies and minds while still savoring the pleasures of dining out.

One of the key aspects of making healthy choices when eating out is being aware of portion sizes. Restaurants often serve large portions, which can lead to overeating.

It's important to listen to your body's hunger and satiety cues, and opt for smaller portions or share a meal with a friend to manage portion control.

Another crucial factor is making informed menu choices. Many restaurants now provide nutritional information such as calorie counts and ingredient lists. Take advantage of this information to select options that align with your nutritional goals. Look for dishes that feature lean proteins, whole grains, and an abundance of fruits and vegetables. Choosing grilled or steamed options over fried or creamy dishes can also significantly reduce the overall calorie and fat intake.

Being mindful of hidden sugars and sodium is crucial. Many sauces, dressings, and condiments used in restaurants contain excessive amounts of added sugars and sodium, which can be detrimental to women's health. Opt for healthier alternatives or ask for these items on the side, allowing you to control the amount you consume.

Maintaining a balanced diet when eating out can be challenging. Prioritize nutrient-dense foods and aim to include all essential food groups. Don't be afraid to customize your order, asking for substitutions or modifications that align with your dietary needs. For example, you can request salad dressings on the side or substitute fries with steamed vegetables.

Remember that eating out should be a pleasurable experience. Indulging in your favorite dishes occasionally is perfectly fine. However, it's essential to strike a balance and make conscious choices most of the time. Enjoy your meal, savor every bite, and focus on the social aspect of dining out rather than solely on the food.

By incorporating these strategies into your eating-out routine, you can navigate the world of dining out with confidence and prioritize your health and well-being. Making mindful choices when eating out will not only ensure proper nutrition but also empower women to take control of their bodies and minds, ultimately leading to optimal health and vitality.

CHAPTER 10: SUSTAINING LONG-TERM NUTRITIONAL SUCCESS

The Power of Habit Formation

In our fast-paced modern world, we often struggle to maintain healthy eating habits. The constant bombardment of advertisements for unhealthy foods and the convenience of processed meals can make it challenging to prioritize our nutrition. However, by understanding the power of habit formation, women can take control of their eating choices and nourish their bodies and minds.

Habits are powerful behaviors that are deeply ingrained in our daily lives. They can either work for us or against

us for nutrition and healthy eating. External factors, such as stress, emotions, and social situations, can influence the development of many of our eating habits. Understanding this, we can identify the habits that are hindering our optimal nutrition and replace them with healthier alternatives.

One of the first steps in habit formation is self-awareness. Women need to assess their current eating habits and identify any patterns that might be detrimental to their health. This could include mindless snacking, emotional eating, or reliance on processed foods. Once you recognize these habits, addressing them and making positive changes becomes easier.

The next step is to set clear goals and create a plan for implementing new habits. For example, if mindless snacking is an issue, women can establish designated snack times and choose healthier options, like fruits or nuts. Planning meals and having a well-stocked pantry with nutritious ingredients can also make it easier to resist the temptation of processed convenience foods.

Accountability is crucial in habit formation. Women can seek support from friends, and family, or even join online communities that share similar nutrition goals. Sharing progress, challenges, and successes with others can

provide motivation and help maintain consistency in healthy eating habits.

Another powerful tool is the concept of habit stacking. This involves attaching a new habit to an existing one. For instance, if a woman wants to incorporate more water consumption into her routine, she can make it a habit to drink a glass of water before each meal or after brushing her teeth. By linking the new habit to an existing one, it becomes easier to remember and incorporate.

It's important to remember that habit formation takes time and patience. Setbacks or slips should not discourage women-ups, but view them as opportunities to learn and grow. With each positive habit formed, women can experience the transformative power of optimal nutrition, not only benefiting their bodies but also nourishing their minds for a healthier and more fulfilling lifestyle.

In conclusion, the power of habit formation can be a significant change for women seeking optimal nutrition and healthy eating habits. By recognizing and replacing detrimental habits, setting clear goals, seeking support, and using techniques like habit stacking, women can take control of their eating choices and nourish their bodies and minds for a vibrant and balanced life.

STAYING MOTIVATED AND OVERCOMING SETBACKS

In our journey toward optimal nutrition and overall well-being, it's important to acknowledge that setbacks are a natural part of the process. As women, we often face unique challenges in nutrition and healthy eating. From juggling multiple responsibilities to dealing with hormonal fluctuations, it's easy to lose motivation and succumb to setbacks. However, by adopting the right mindset and implementing effective strategies, we can stay motivated and overcome any obstacles that come our way.

One of the key factors in staying motivated is understanding our personal goals and reasons for embarking on this journey. Take some time to reflect on why optimal nutrition is important to you. Whether it's to have more energy, maintain a healthy weight, or prevent chronic

diseases, connecting with your deeper motivations will fuel your determination to stay on track.

Another powerful tool for staying motivated is surrounding yourself with a supportive community. Seek like-minded women who are also passionate about nutrition and healthy eating. Join online forums, attend local meetups, or even start a book club to discuss your progress, share tips, and encourage others. Having a support system can make all the difference during challenging times.

When setbacks occur, it's crucial to approach them as opportunities for learning and growth. Analyze what went wrong, identify triggers or patterns, and brainstorm strategies to prevent similar setbacks in the future. Remember, progress is not always linear, and setbacks are a natural part of the journey toward optimal nutrition.

Self-compassion is essential when overcoming setbacks. Beating yourself over a slip-up or indulgence will only lead to negative emotions and further setbacks. Instead, acknowledge your humanity and practice forgiveness. Treat setbacks as temporary detours and use them as motivation to recommit to your goals.

Finally, maintaining motivation and overcoming setbacks require consistency and accountability. Set realistic, achievable goals and create a plan to track your pro

gress. Whether it's keeping a food journal, using a fitness app, or scheduling regular check-ins with a nutritionist or accountability partner, find a system that works for you.

In conclusion, staying motivated and overcoming setbacks is crucial in our pursuit of optimal nutrition and overall well-being as women. By understanding our motivations, building a support system, practicing self-compassion, and maintaining consistency, we can navigate through setbacks and continue on our journey toward a nourished body and mind. Remember, the path to optimal nutrition is not always easy, but with determination and resilience, we can overcome any obstacle that stands in our way.

BUILDING A SUPPORTIVE COMMUNITY FOR LASTING RESULTS

In our journey towards optimal nutrition and a healthy lifestyle, it is crucial to recognize the power of the community. As women, we often find strength in coming together, supporting one another, and sharing our experiences. By building a supportive community, we can enhance our chances of achieving lasting results and create a positive impact on our overall well-being.

Nutrition and healthy eating for women can sometimes feel overwhelming and isolating. We face unique challenges, including hormonal fluctuations, societal pressures, and busy lifestyles. However, by establishing a supportive community, we can overcome these obstacles and thrive together.

The first step in building a supportive community is finding like-minded individuals who share similar goals and interests. Seek local groups, online forums, or social media communities that focus on nutrition and healthy eating for women. Surrounding yourself with individuals who have similar aspirations will provide motivation, encouragement, and a safe space to share experiences and seek advice.

Within this community, it is essential to foster an environment of inclusivity, respect, and empathy. Each woman's journey is unique, and we must celebrate and support one another's accomplishments, no matter how big or small. By creating a non-judgmental atmosphere, we can inspire one another to make positive changes and maintain healthy habits.

Regular communication is key to nurturing a supportive community. Organize regular meet-ups, whether they are virtual or in-person, to discuss challenges, share tips and recipes, and offer encouragement. Consider hosting potluck dinners or cooking workshops to foster a sense of camaraderie and inspire creativity in the kitchen.

Besides connecting with like-minded individuals, it is essential to seek guidance from professionals within the

community. Nutritionists, dietitians, and other experts can provide valuable insights and personalized advice to help us navigate our unique nutritional needs as women. Their expertise can help us make informed decisions and achieve optimal results.

Building a supportive community goes beyond sharing nutrition tips; it extends to other aspects of our lives. Encourage open conversations about mental health, self-care, and body image. By addressing these topics, we can break down stigmas, support one another through challenging times, and promote holistic well-being.

Thank you for taking the time in reading this book. I feel it is important in building a supportive community. It

is vital for women seeking optimal nutrition and healthy eating habits. By surrounding ourselves with like-minded individuals, fostering inclusivity and respect, and seeking guidance from professionals, we can create an environment that empowers us to achieve lasting results. Together, we can nourish our bodies and minds, celebrate our successes, and uplift one another in our journey toward optimal health.